Zoltan Ron

Natural
Alternatives
to
Vaccination

Be informed about
- **the side effects and dangers of vaccinations**
- **immune-boosting strategies**
- **your right to decide**

alive books

Vancouver
Canada

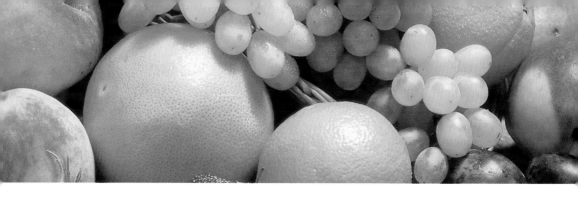

Contents

All About Vaccination Alternatives

Note: Conversions in this book (from imperial to metric) are not exact. They have been rounded to the nearest measurement for convenience. Exact measurements are given in imperial. The recipes in this book are by no means to be taken as therapeutic. They simply promote the philosophy of both the author and *alive* books in relation to whole foods, health and nutrition, while incorporating the practical advice given by the author in the first section of the book.

Immune-Boosting Recipes

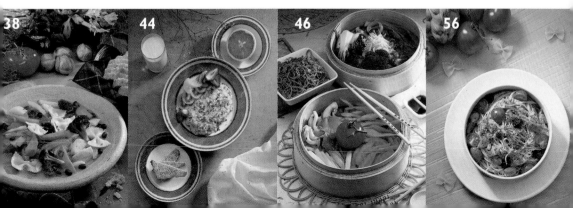

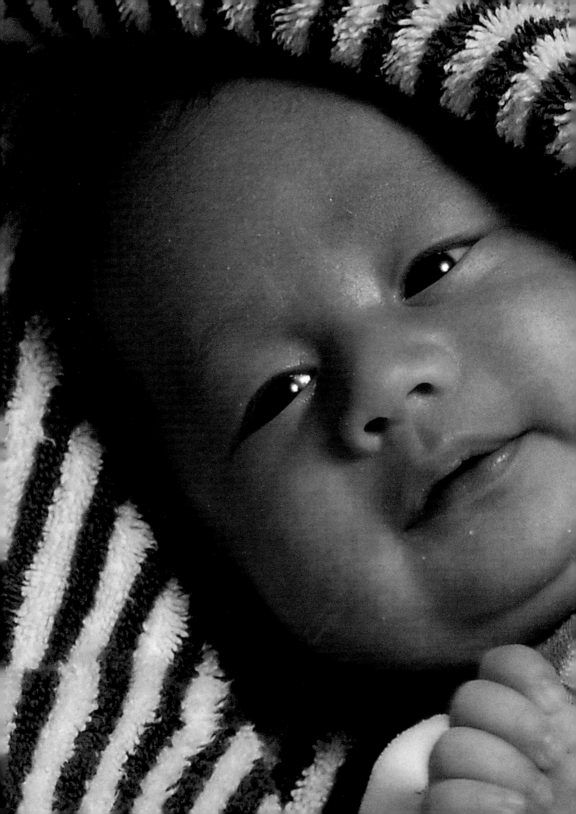

All About Vaccination Alternatives

Many, myself included, question the ethics and wisdom of sacrificing even a small number of children in the belief that society will be free of an ever-expanding list of infectious diseases. A growing body of anecdotal and scientific evidence indicates that vaccines may not be as safe or as effective as claimed.

— Zoltan Rona, MD

The antivaccination movement is no longer a cult.

It may surprise you to know that about one-third of the four million babies born in the United States and Canada every year remain unvaccinated at age two. This "failure to vaccinate," as it is termed by vaccination proponents, is largely due to concerned parents, who, after considerable personal research, consciously choose to forgo or change how their children receive medical vaccinations. Authority figures in the medical profession and the government claim that such decisions are based on dangerously erroneous conclusions, on ignorance, poverty, conspiracy paranoia, and constitute a hidden form of child abuse.

Today, the antivaccination movement is no longer a cult. Led by a new wave of respected scientists and health care professionals, the unvaccinated population is expanding at a remarkable rate. Many popular books have been written on the subject, including the shocking best seller *The Medical Mafia* by Dr. Guylaine Lanctot (Here's The Key Inc., 1995), a brave Canadian physician who lost her medical license in Quebec for daring to advise the public against conventional immunizations.

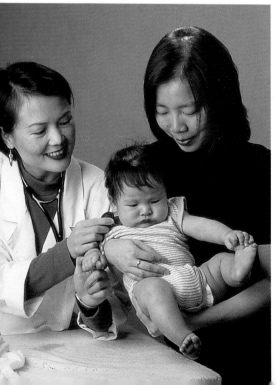

While freedom of speech and expression may be enshrined in the Canadian Charter of Rights and Freedoms, it does not, apparently, apply to the medical profession.

The following pages are not intended to sway your opinion one way or another about conventional vaccinations. They will, however, provide information that will clarify why natural alternatives may be preferable to conventional vaccinations. I am mainly concerned about the safety of vaccines. As a physician, it is part of my training and belief that it is better to do nothing than to do harm. And in the case of vaccinations, I question whether the benefits really outweigh the risks.

While much has been written criticizing medical vaccines, there has never been a book about reasonably safe and effective alternatives. As you will soon read, there is a great deal one can do to protect against infectious disease with nutrition, vitamins, herbs and homeopathy. Much attention has been placed on supportive scientific documentation for these alternatives, and readers are encouraged to look up the many references provided so as to more fully understand these options.

Many, myself included, question the ethics and wisdom of sacrificing even a small number of children in the belief that society will be free of an ever-expanding list of infectious diseases. A growing body of anecdotal and scientific evidence indicates that vaccines may not be as safe or as effective as claimed. In fact, studies are increasingly pointing to the conclusion that vaccines represent a dangerous assault on the immune system, leading to autoimmune diseases like multiple sclerosis, lupus, juvenile onset diabetes, fibromyalgia and chronic fatigue syndrome, as well as previously rare disorders like brain cancer, childhood leukemia, sudden infant death syndrome (SIDS), autism and asthma.

If you haven't made a firm decision about vaccinations, I strongly recommend that you read what various experts have to say and formulate your own opinions. Do not rely solely on the advice of your doctor, but do ask your doctor about the risks and possible side effects, and then complement this information with what has been written on this subject.

There is a great deal one can do to protect against infectious disease with nutrition, vitamins, herbs and homeopathy.

Why Many Say "No" To Vaccinations . . .

Threats, admonitions and medical ostracisms have, to date, failed to win back the millions opting out of the medical vaccination paradigm. However, anyone who decides against vaccinating their children is going against conventional medical wisdom and is likely to hear a message that goes something like this:

"*The Centers for Disease Control (CDC) and the Food and Drug Administration (FDA) are not aware of any alternative methods to safely and effectively prevent these serious infectious diseases long term. Some individuals and groups propose that 'natural' substances that 'boost' a child's immune*

The greatest threat of childhood diseases lies in the dangerous and ineffectual efforts made to prevent them through mass immunization.
– Robert Mendelsohn, MD

system are an alternative to vaccination. However, many people with healthy immune systems have died from diseases that could have been prevented with vaccination . . . A child left unvaccinated is left to battle a disease organism without the help of the antibodies that the child's immune system would have developed through vaccination. While many unvaccinated children will survive such a battle, many will do so only after suffering severe complications that may lead to disabilities.

The American Academy of Pediatrics, The American Academy of Family Physicians, and the CDC recommend that children routinely be vaccinated against ten serious diseases."

(compiled from CDC and FDA documents, 1998)

These are strong words. Yet, for a variety of reasons they are unheeded by millions. Medical vaccines have come under fire in the past decade. A growing number of parents and doctors worry that vaccines can cause illness and death in numbers much larger than generally acknowledged by pediatric and government authorities.

Increasingly, parental fears are fueled by the fact that the United States government has set up the Vaccine Injury Compensation Program, which, in the first five years paid over half a billion dollars for vaccine-related injuries and deaths. Added to this concern are government figures showing that less than 10 percent of doctors even report vaccine problems. Do parents really know if the benefits of immunization outweigh the risks?

Vaccines Currently Recommended by American and Canadian Pediatricians

Diphtheria, Pertussis, Tetanus (DPT; combined) to be given at two, four, six, fifteen months and again at four to six years of age, then every ten years thereafter.

Hepatitis B to be given shortly after birth, and at two and six months of age.

Polio at two, four, fifteen months and again at four to six years of age.

Haemophilus influenzae type B at two, four, six and fifteen months.

Measles, Mumps, Rubella (MMR; combined) at fifteen months and again at four to six years of age.

Chickenpox anytime after twelve months of age.

Dogma vs. Fact . . . .

> There is no credible scientific data to demonstrate that the injection of multiple antigens into a baby, particularly a baby under the age of one year, is safe and effective. There is no credible scientific evidence to negate the hypothesis that vaccines cause immediate or delayed damage to the immune system as well as neurological disorders . . .
>
> – Stephen Marini, PhD

Mainstream doctors regard vaccinations as dogma, never to be questioned or refused for any reason. This dogma is enforced by various government agencies that blindly follow the dictates of the medical and pharmaceutical lobbies. Like antibiotics, cancer chemotherapy, the annual physical, mammograms and Pap tests, the validity of vaccinations is on the same emotional footing as motherhood and apple pie.

Vaccines are the only product sold for profit in North America that carry the risk of injury or death and yet are practically forced upon every healthy citizen. Until the late 1980s, few questioned the wisdom of this lucrative pharmaceutical enterprise. Regardless of the scare tactics and rhetoric, the fact is that parents in both Canada and the United States have the legal right to refuse vaccinations for themselves and their children.

Every province in Canada and every state in the US allows exemptions to compulsory vaccinations for religious, personal or philosophical beliefs. Anyone telling you otherwise is misinformed or, whether they mean to or not, are promoting a particular belief system.

The US and Canadian governments, supported by questionable studies and with the financial assistance of vaccine manufacturers, promote compulsory vaccination of healthy children. According to those who have analyzed the studies, pro-vaccination papers are statistically flawed and illogical. Moreover, studies designed to look at the long-term safety of vaccines are virtually non-existent.

The fact is that vaccines can be dangerous. Information regarding the safety and efficacy of immunization is not readily available to the general public. The powers that be are not likely to freely

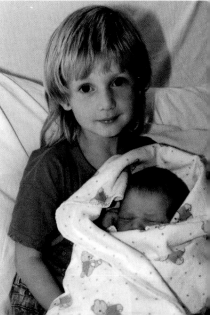

admit to the negative aspects of vaccines for the simple reason that there are millions of dollars and great political power tied up in the promotion of immunizations. So, it is up to the individual to question the dogma and probe for the truth.

How Vaccines Work Against the Body . . . .

> It is dangerously misleading, and indeed, the exact opposite of truth, to claim that a vaccine makes us "immune" or protects against disease. In fact, it only drives the disease deeper into the interior and causes us to harbor it chronically, with the result that our responses to it become progressively weaker and show less tendency to heal or restore themselves spontaneously.
>
> – Richard Moskowitz, MD

Traditional Chinese medical practitioners believe that measles, mumps and chicken pox are beneficial childhood diseases that boost immunity and help rid the body of harmful poisons. And there are doctors, myself included, who believe that childhood illnesses are important to the maturation and development of the immune system. A healthy immune system defends against allergies, infections, asthma, eczema and even cancer. Suppressing normal childhood illnesses could very well backfire on the population as a whole.

Common childhood illnesses are seen by some to protect against more serious, life-threatening conditions. This theory has to do with how the immune system responds to an invader. If the infection with measles happens at a time when there are already antibodies against the measles virus present (i.e., within the first few months after birth in the child who has been immunized) the immune system cannot react fully to the infection, giving the virus the chance to become persistent, and to develop later as an autoimmune disease or other chronic allergic problem.

There is a school of thought that measles, mumps, rubella (German measles) and chicken pox, which enter the body through the mucous membranes, serve a necessary and positive purpose in challenging and strengthening the immune system of these membranes. In contrast, the respective vaccines of these diseases are injected by needle directly into the system of the child, thereby bypassing the mucosal immune system. As a result, mucosal immunity remains relatively weak and stunted in many children, complications which may be linked to the rapid increase in asthma and eczema now being seen.

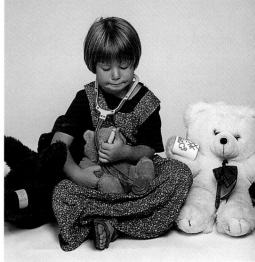

Importantly, vaccinations may temporarily lower immune function. This concern is based on research that found that T-cell (white blood cell) ratios fell to low levels for up to two weeks after tetanus booster doses in apparently healthy persons.

Moreover, it is a common observation made by parents and clinical practitioners of many types that children are more likely to suffer ear infections just after vaccinations. I have certainly noted this in my practice.

Vaccinations Can Cause Disease . . . .

> The best immunity is natural immunity. It is normally found in 80 to 90 percent of the population under the age of fifteen. Because the contamination of a person by an illness mobilizes the body's defense systems, natural immunization goes hand in hand with being sick. Contamination from vaccines, on the other hand, short-circuits all the body's first line of defenses. Artificial immunization adds to the disorder.
> – Guylaine Lanctot, MD

There is ample evidence, if one looks for it, of serious problems with vaccines. It is not the focus of this book to detail the many examples of the ineffectiveness of vaccines, or the negative reactions, or the deaths as a result of immunizations. However, following are some examples of immunization incidents, which will give you an idea of some of the problems inherent in vaccines:

• Of the 145 children who died of crib death (Sudden Infant Death Syndrome or SIDS) in Los Angeles County from 1979 to 1980, more than one-third had received the diphtheria-tetanus-pertussis (DTP) vaccine less than a month earlier. These sids cases were significantly more than expected for a vaccine purported to be "safe and effective."

- In 1988 the British National Childhood Encephalopathy Study (NCES) in Great Britain concluded that there was a relationship between neurological illness and DTP immunization in children aged two months to thirty-six months. Children who experienced a serious acute reaction to the DTP vaccine were found to be at risk for later chronic nervous system dysfunction.
- It is a matter of public record that Jonas Salk, inventor of the injected polio vaccine, testified to a Senate sub-committee that the oral polio vaccine has caused most of the polio outbreaks since 1961.
- The Ohio Department of Health reported that 2,720 children developed measles in 1989 despite the fact that close to three-quarters of the cases occurred in previously vaccinated children. The US Centers for Disease Control and Prevention (CDC) even reported measles outbreaks in a documented 100 percent vaccinated population. According to the CDC, among school-aged children, measles outbreaks have occurred in schools with vaccination levels greater than 98 percent. These outbreaks have occurred in all parts of the country, including areas that had not reported measles for years. Half of the reported pertussis cases in Ohio from 1987 to 1991 occurred in children who were vaccinated.

Is Vaccination Necessary?

Medical literature documents a surprisingly high incidence of vaccine failures for measles, mumps, polio, small pox, and influenza in vaccinated populations.

For most diseases for which vaccines are given, disease and death rates had already fallen dramatically prior to widespread vaccination. For example, mortality from diphtheria was already reduced to six per 100,000 children in 1940–before the introduction of the vaccine. Mortality from measles was already less than one per 100,000 infected in 1955, eight years before the vaccine was produced. In both cases, the diseases had already become less deadly before the introduction of vaccines.

The decreasing incidence of childhood diseases parallels improved sanitation and hygienic practices rather than vaccination programs. Prior to vaccinations, infectious disease deaths in the US and England declined steadily by an average of about 80 percent during this century, with measles mortality declining by 97 percent. Poverty, crowded conditions, poor nutrition, lack of access to medical care and unsanitary conditions are far more likely to contribute to the development and spread of disease than the absence of a vaccine.

Even the most outspoken vaccine advocates admit that shots are not 100 percent effective. Measles epidemics in populations with an immunization rate of close to 100 percent are not uncommon. Fife, Scotland, despite a vaccination density of 96 percent, experienced a measles epidemic in 1991-92, followed shortly by outbreaks of measles in other parts of the country, even though there was a high density of MMR vaccination.

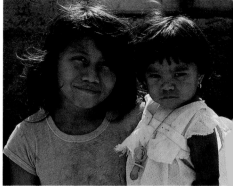

Common childhood illnesses are seen by some to protect against more serious, life threatening conditions.

Medical literature documents a surprisingly high incidence of vaccine failures for measles, mumps, polio, small pox, influenza and numerous other contagious diseases in vaccinated populations. One of the theories as to why this occurs is that vaccination results in immune suppression, which then creates an increased susceptibility to infections.

Dangerous Additives . . . .

A major cause of the Roman Empire's decline, after six centuries of world dominance, was the replacement of stone aqueducts by lead pipes for the transport and supply of drinking water. Roman engineers, the best in the world, turned their fellow citizens into neurological cripples. Today our own "best and brightest," with the best of intentions, achieve the same end through childhood vaccination programs yielding the modern scourges of hyperactivity, learning disabilities, autism, appetite disorders and impulsive violence.

– Harris L. Coulter, PhD

Vaccines contain a long list of potentially dangerous additives that are being injected into two-, four- and six-month old infants whose immune systems are not fully developed.
The chemicals found in standard vaccinations are blamed by some experts for many adverse reactions. These reactions may occur immediately or they may not make themselves known until years later.

Vaccine Ingredients . . . .

The following are some of the ingredients found in vaccines:

Thimerosal - A preservative containing mercury that has been used as an additive in vaccines since the 1930s. While no severe, life-threatening reactions have been reported as a direct result of thimerosal, there is concern about this additive because of recent findings concerning the toxicity of mercury to the nervous and immune systems. In addition, with children now receiving a dozen or more injections of mercury-containing vaccines, even the Centers for Disease Control has raised some serious doubts and concerns about the safety of this additive.

On October 22, 1998, the American FDA banned thimerosal from any over-the-counter drug preparations because "safety and efficacy have not been established for the ingredients . . ." Despite this ban, thimerosal continues to be present in vaccines given to Canadian and American children.

In June 1999 the FDA revealed that infants who receive multiple doses of vaccines containing thimerosal would be exposed to total amounts of mercury that exceeded some federal guidelines. After public pressure, on July 7, 1999, the American Academy of Pediatrics (AAP) and the US Public Health Service (PHS) released a joint statement acknowledging the dangers of thimerosal. Despite these facts, vaccines containing mercury continue to be used by physicians who justify their use by minimizing the dangers of mercury.

Formaldehyde - The toxicity of this cancer-causing chemical should be of great concern to parents, especially when infants and children receive over a dozen different needles containing this substance before they reach school age. Formaldehyde can cause allergic reactions on both an immediate and delayed hypersensitivity basis, leading to potentially chronic immune system problems. According to the US Poisons Information Center: "There is no acceptable safe amount of formaldehyde if being injected into a living human body. It is a toxic substance and should be avoided at all costs."

Sulfite - Sodium metabisulfite is a preservative also found in many foods and some alcoholic beverages. Large oral doses of sulfites can cause shortness of breath, wheezing, diarrhea, vomiting, cramps and dizziness.

Monosodium glutamate (MSG) - MSG is a stabilizer known to cause adverse reactions in some people. In fact, there is a condition known as "Chinese Restaurant Syndrome" that causes nausea, vomiting, dizziness, headache and diarrhea as a direct result of eating foods containing MSG.

Aluminum gels - These substances are found in a wide range of vaccines, and have been associated with reactions like erythema and subcutaneous nodules. Aluminum is a neurotoxin and has been linked to Alzheimer's as well as other nervous system disorders.

Antibiotics - While penicillin is no longer added to vaccines due to its strong allergic potential, manufacturers routinely use similar antibiotics to prevent bacterial contamination. Even trace doses of these drugs may cause severe allergies in susceptible people.

Foreign genetic material - Humans can get diseases from monkey and other animal tissue used in the production of vaccines. Vaccines such as MMR and polio are attenuated in living organisms or cell cultures (kidney cell cultures of monkeys). The rubella portion of the MMR vaccine is cultured on the cell-lines of aborted fetuses.

It is technologically impossible to exclude all possible risk of vaccine contamination. One such risk is the infestation of the sample by various viruses that cause deadly diseases and that have such a long latency period that a causal connection is almost impossible to detect. A live vaccine produced by conventional procedures can become a carrier of unknown genetic modifications or mutations—any number of viruses, for example.

Animals that are contaminated with a virus and whose cells are used to make a vaccine can inadvertently transfer that virus. Once injected into an infant, this virus could stay dormant for many years, only to surface at age forty as brain cancer. A virus can infect any cell in the body and cause malignant transformation: In other words, a virus can change a healthy cell into one that is malignant (cancerous).

Link to Autoimmune Diseases? . . . . . .

Doctors and governments push full-scale immunization despite incomplete knowledge of what vaccines do to the immune system. For example, it has been frequently observed that antibody levels do not go hand in hand with immunity to the disease for which the vaccination is given. The potential disease-provoking properties of a vaccine are largely unknown, and no one has been able to guarantee that autoimmune disease is not the end result of damage caused by vaccines.

A causal connection between vaccinations and the onset of autoimmune disease remains to be proven. However, several authors have argued that conditions such as juvenile rheumatoid arthritis could be the body's reaction to foreign pathogens contained in vaccines. The body's immune system is designed to defend against infectious disease-causing organisms. When presented with a foreign pathogen, the immune system mobilizes to fight off the "enemy."

Over time the immune system comes to "memorize" a number of invaders, and, can therefore respond quickly to an intruder. However, certain foreign substances–vaccines, for example–may have a similar structure as some body tissue; as a result, the antibodies that are produced to attack the pathogens in the vaccine could also lead to the immune system attacking body tissue with a similar structure. It is this lack of differentiation between the body's own tissue and foreign cells that leads to autoimmune diseases.

Vaccines and Childhood Allergies . . . . .

Hay fever, asthma, eczema, chronic fatigue syndrome, fibromyalgia, multiple sclerosis and psoriasis have all been associated with food and chemical allergies. Many pediatricians blame the rising incidence of these allergic conditions on the early ingestion of allergenic foods. The early introduction of allergens has been documented to increase the incidence of chronic allergic illness.

Despite such reports, children at a very early age are aggressively exposed to foreign proteins (allergens) in the form of immunizations. It doesn't make sense that doctors on the one hand advise parents to avoid early childhood contact with allergens, and then, on the other hand, promote vaccinations that expose children to allergens.

Given the growing severity of immune diseases in children, especially asthma, shouldn't there first be studies aimed at the connection between immunizations and subsequent immune system impairment? Conventional medical authorities demand proof of the safety and efficacy of natural remedies before they are to be recommended to children: Why isn't the same proof demanded for vaccinations?

The Flu Shot . . . .

The flu vaccine, consumed faithfully by the public without question each year, is not without problems. The vaccine contains formaldehyde, a known cancer-causing agent. It also contains the preservative thimerosal, a derivative of mercury, a known neurotoxin linked to brain damage and autoimmune diseases. Aluminum is yet another flu vaccine ingredient. Mercury and aluminum are two toxic heavy metals that have been associated with an increased incidence of Alzheimer's disease.

Outbreaks of the flu still occur despite widespread use of the recommended flu vaccine.

Side effects reported as a result of the flu vaccine include fever, general malaise, muscle pain, hives, allergic asthma, respiratory tract infections, gastrointestinal problems, eye problems, abnormal blood pressure and other circulatory abnormalities. Moreover, those with a severe allergy to eggs are advised against the flu shot because the flu vaccine is propagated on chicken embryo cells.

The influenza epidemic that hit North America so strongly in January 2000 was the worst in five years. Of interest is the fact that a large percentage of the elderly who contracted the flu did so despite having had their flu shots. One nursing home in Toronto recorded thirty-two cases of the flu; of those individuals who became ill, thirty-one had been vaccinated for the flu the previous month!

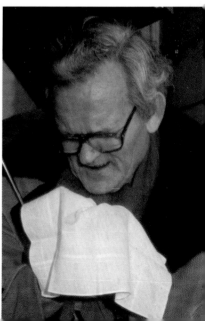

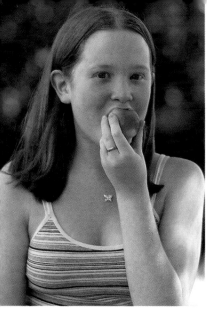

Fresh, organic fruit and vegetables are part of an immune-enhancing diet.

Outbreaks of the flu still occur despite widespread use of the recommended flu vaccine. The excuse made for such immunization failures is that the wrong virus was predicted for use in the flu vaccine.

The actual composition of the flu vaccine is based on an educated guess made by a consensus of about thirty public-health experts. These "experts" meet annually with the FDA in the US to predict which specific strains of influenza will invade the country in the coming year. If this sounds unscientific to you, it's because it is. As a result the flu vaccine's effectiveness rate is only about 20 percent.

Vaccination proponents are at a loss to explain such figures. They are also at a loss to explain why it is that so many unvaccinated individuals do not get the flu. I would suggest that it has to do with an individual's immune system.

A healthy immune system is a strong defense against disease. Even if you, or your child, has been vaccinated by the conventional route, there is a great deal you can and ought to do to enhance the immune system naturally. There are no magic bullets, conventional or otherwise, that will guarantee freedom from infectious illness. However, your immunity—and therefore your resistance to infectious disease—can be greatly improved by following the basic diet and lifestyle guidelines outlined in this book.

Healthy Travel Without Vaccinations

One should embark on an immune-enhancing diet before embarking on a trip It is possible to have a healthy vacation abroad if you take some basic precautions. In particular, pay careful attention to food and water sanitation. And watch what you eat and drink.

Avoid tap water. Use ozonated bottled water, or add 20 drops of 3 percent hydrogen peroxide, or a liquid oxygen supplement like Aerobic Oxygen, or add ¼ teaspoon of Bioxy Cleanse to each 8 ounces of untreated water.

Avoid meat if possible. Parasites are found in highest concentrations in beef, chicken, lamb, pork and pork products (bacon, ham, hot dogs, cold cuts) and fish. Sushi may contain the larvae of several species of parasitic worms. If you must eat animal products, ensure that they are well cooked and that you take digestive enzyme supplements.

It is important to realize that one has the legal right to refuse "mandatory" travel vaccinations.

There Are Alternatives . . . .

A large number of reputable scientists point to the fact that there is no proof that germs cause disease in the first place. They argue that the foundation upon which vaccination theory is built is flawed. It is a proven fact that up to 90 percent of the decrease in infectious disease occurred before the introduction of vaccines or antibiotics. Scarlet fever, for example, has disappeared despite the fact that there has never been a vaccine or treatment for it. Given this, it would certainly make sense to treat the "diseased tissue"–the biological terrain, so to speak. The approach should be to strengthen the body's immune defenses with diet and lifestyle changes so that the "germs" are rendered impotent.

> If I could live my life over again, I would devote it to proving that germs seek their natural habitat–diseased tissue–rather than being the cause of the diseased tissue.
> – Rudolph Virchow, founder of cellular medicine.

While there is good anecdotal and observational evidence to support vaccine alternatives, there is very little hard scientific proof that any of the non-conventional approaches work to prevent childhood or adult illnesses. Neither conventional nor alternative immunization strategies can offer 100 percent protection, and no one has ever published acceptable comparison studies concluding that an alternative approach is superior to the mainstream or vice versa.

However, after reviewing the alternative medical literature, several approaches stand out as the best ways of immunizing both children and adults naturally. The more of the following suggestions that are incorporated into your health regime, the greater the chances of successfully preventing life-threatening illnesses.

- Sugar-free, immune-enhancing diet
- Bovine colostrum
- Probiotics
- Natural interferon boosters
- Other natural immunizing agents
- Homeopathic nosodes

Breastfeeding–A Good Start . . . .

The best defense against infection and disease is the body's natural immune system. And the best way to kick-start a baby's immune system is through breast-feeding. A breastfed baby

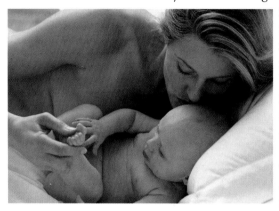

receives antibodies through the mother's milk, as well as all the nutrients needed for the first six months of their life. Much of the benefit of breastfeeding is derived from colostrum, the mammary fluid secreted the first few days after delivery.

Colustrum provides newborns with protection against bacteria and viruses through its content of immune factors (antibodies and natural antibiotics) as well as essential nutrients including various growth factors, vitamins, minerals and hormones. These can help prevent a variety of problems, including ear infections and diarrhea. The benefits of colostrum can also be had through bovine colostrum, a nutritional supplement (discussed in more detail later on).

Immunity can be enhanced and food allergies can be minimized or prevented if solid foods and beverages are introduced to the breast-fed infant properly. Infants should not be fed cow's milk, wheat, oranges, eggs, honey or chocolate for the first year of life. Other foods can be introduced gradually after six months of age.

High protein and highly allergenic foods should be introduced, ideally, after twenty-one months of age. These include egg, milk, citrus, wheat, corn, shellfish, nuts and foods containing yeast. It is best to introduce one new food at a time. A new food can be introduced every four days, noting such reactions as sneezing, runny nose, rash, irritability, diarrhea or vomiting. If a food causes any of these reactions it should be avoided. Ideally, well-tolerated foods should be rotated on a four-day basis so as to minimize sensitization that often occurs when foods are eaten repetitively.

Optimizing the Immune System . . .

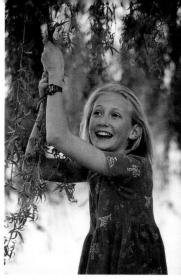

The immune system can be optimized to prevent infection, minimize the impact of allergies and protect against disease. If the dietary changes described below cause too much weight loss increase the intake of legumes like chick peas, pinto beans, navy beans as well as squash, fruits, avocados, rice, yams and fermented soy products.

It goes without saying that for optimal health one should not smoke, and should limit alcohol and drug consumption as much as possible. It is also important to get regular exercise, daily sunshine, rest and sleep since all these lifestyle factors affect immunity. Stress reduction is also important since stress will cause an adverse effect on the adrenal glands, which manufacture hormones that augment immunity.

Immune-Enhancing Supplements for Healthy Children
Cod liver oil: 1 tablespoon daily (a mint flavored product is palatable)
Probiotics (broad spectrum): 1 teaspoon daily (powdered acidophilus and bifidum products are available)
Bovine colostrums: 500 milligram capsule twice daily
Larch arabinogalactan: 1 teaspoon daily (it tastes rather bitter and is best taken in juice)
Vitamin C with bioflavonoids: 500 milligrams daily
Green drink containing wheat grass: 1 teaspoon in water or juice daily
The above supplements are available in health food stores.

The immune-enhancing diet that is described here applies equally to infants, children and adults. An immune-enhancing diet employs the following basic approaches:

Eat more organic vegetables

Organic vegetables are free of dangerous pesticides and contain two to five times more nutrients than non-organic vegetables. They also taste much better. If you cannot obtain organic vegetables, you can rinse non-organic produce in a sink of cold water with a half-cup of distilled white vinegar for thirty minutes. This will remove much of the pesticides.

Practically all vegetables have something beneficial to offer, including vitamins, minerals, essential fats, phyto-chemicals and fiber. Eat a wide variety, provided you are not allergic to them and they do not cause gas or intestinal problems. Vegetables are best

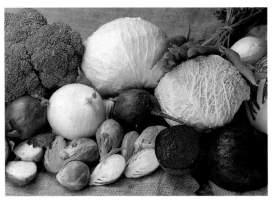

eaten raw; however, it is certainly acceptable to lightly steam them until the body gets used to the roughage. Not all vegetables are therapeutic or offer immune system benefits: iceberg lettuce, for example, has minimal nutritional value. Better alternatives are kale, Swiss chard, collards and spinach. Carrots are fine in small amounts (one medium-sized carrot daily), but they are high in sugar and provitamin A, which, in excess, can lead to low blood sugar reactions and a yellow-orange discoloration of the skin from too much carotene.

Vegetables that can be eaten in unlimited amounts are red and green leaf lettuce, romaine lettuce, broccoli, Chinese cabbage, bok choy, fennel, radishes, green onions, endive, escarole, celery, cucumbers, cauliflower, broccoli, squash, zucchini, Brussels sprouts, turnips, dandelion greens, green and red cabbage, Jerusalem artichokes, kohlrabi, cilantro and parsley.

Drink more water and fresh vegetable juices

Water is the beverage of choice, preferably bottled spring water, although reverse osmosis filtered water is acceptable. Drink at least eight glasses of water a day. Avoid buying water in plastic containers from your grocery store as the plastic transfers far too many chemicals into the water. The five-gallon containers from the water companies are made of a much harder plastic and don't impart anywhere near as many chemicals to the water as the one- to three-liter bottles.

Avoid drinking tap water that contains harmful chemicals like chlorine and, in some cities, fluoride. Avoid softened or distilled water as it contains no minerals, has the wrong ionization, pH, polarization and oxidation potentials, and tends to drain the body of minerals.

Freshly juiced vegetables are a convenient way of getting concentrated vitamins, minerals and other healthy nutrients–especially vitamin C and bioflavonoids. Avoid coffee unless it is organic, and even then limit its intake. Coffee in large amounts (more than two cups daily) acts as a diuretic, causing the loss of important trace minerals. Green tea or herbal teas are a better option.

Eat more healthy fats

Healthy fats provide the omega-3, -6 and -9 essential fatty acids. One of the best sources is hempseed oil. One tablespoon daily will provide the necessary essential fat. If your skin is on the dry side, use more. If your skin turns oily with this supplement, reduce the dose. A combination of fish oils and flax seed oil is an alternative to hempseed oil.

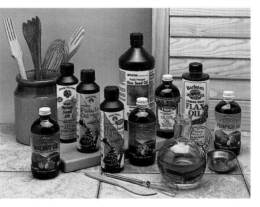

Raw sunflower and pumpkin seeds are also good sources of these fats. Avoid peanuts, peanut butter and peanut oil at all costs. They contain mold and aflatoxin, a known immune suppressor. According to experts in mycology (the study of fungi), no peanut sold in North America is free of aflatoxin, even organic ones. For more information on oils read *Good Fats and Oils* (alive Natural Health Guides, 2000).

Avoid sugar

Sugar impairs immunity and promotes yeast and fungal overgrowth. Sugar in any form suppresses immunity and must be eliminated as much as possible from the diet. Several studies published in medical and scientific journals support this claim.

Avoid hidden sources of refined sugar in things like pop and in most packaged cereals. Limit natural sweeteners such as honey, molasses, fruit juice, maple syrup, cane sugar and lactose. Stevia is a better alternative if you tend to use large amounts of sweetener in beverages or cooking. Artificial sweeteners like aspartame should be avoided because of their many adverse health effects. They are particularly harmful to children.

Avoid trans-fatty acids

Hydrogenated vegetable oils, such as those found in margarines, contain trans-fatty acids, which have been reported to significantly raise the risk of heart disease. Even "partially hydrogenated" products should be considered a poison to your system. Other unsuspected sources of trans-fatty acids are commercially made potato and corn chips, French fries, doughnuts, crackers, cookies, pastries, imitation cheeses, frostings, candies and deep fried foods, particularly those from fast food restaurants. Use olive oil, coconut oil or butter for stir-frying vegetables. Canola oil and corn oil are not recommended.

Butter is an acceptable alternative to margarine provided it is organic (containing none of the pesticides, antibiotics and growth hormones found in commercial brands).

Avoid commercial milk and dairy products

Commercial (pasteurized) dairy products contain traces of hormones, antibiotics and other immune-suppressing chemicals. Raw, unpasteurized milk would be acceptable for most people, but it is not commercially available. Dairy allergy is the most common cause of middle ear infections as well as other frequent or recurrent childhood infections. It has been linked to the development of juvenile diabetes and other autoimmune diseases. Those who do not get enough of these nutrients from non-dairy sources such as greens, fish or seafood may require a calcium and vitamin D supplement.

Avoid fruit juices

Bottled fruit juices, including organic, unsweetened varieties, are high in sugar and usually contaminated with mold. Sugar and mold suppress the immune system.

Avoid pork and most commercial meats

Pork is frequently contaminated with parasites and mold. Moreover, pork is used in labs to culture cancer cells, as it increases their growth. Organic buffalo, venison, chicken, turkey, beef and lamb are better options since they contain no hormones, antibiotics or pesticides. Avoid processed, cured, smoked or dried meats, especially bacon, sausage, salami, ham, hot dogs and luncheon meats. Ground meat products may be contaminated with bacteria and should also be avoided.

Eat local fruit

Limit intake of bananas, oranges, papayas, mangoes, melons and other tropical fruit. They are generally much higher in sugar and are not as easily metabolized by people who live in cold climates.

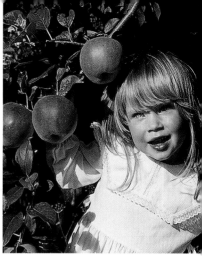

Local fruit is easily metabolized by the body.

The higher the fruit sugar content the higher the level of mold infestation. Thus it is almost impossible to avoid mold if one consumes fruit. Eat local fruit like apples, plums, pears, cherries, blueberries, raspberries and strawberries, all of which are much lower in sugar and mold content. Avoid dried fruits, especially raisins, for the same reasons.

Avoid shellfish

Lobsters, crabs, shrimp and other shellfish are scavengers, frequently contaminated with parasites and viruses that can suppress immunity. They are best eliminated from the diet. Cold-water fish like cod, halibut, salmon, trout and mackerel are better choices.

Use sea salt

Regular table salt is processed and dried at extremely high temperatures, changing the chemical structure of the minerals. Harmful additives and chemicals, including sugar, can be found in typical table salt. Sea salt and sea kelp powder are better alternatives.

Avoid microwave ovens

There is evidence that suggests that microwaves can seriously deplete foods of their enzymes and nutrients while creating radiation byproducts that may cause negative health effects.

All heating causes loss of nutrients, but microwave cooking produces the greatest losses. Steaming, stir-frying and regular convection ovens are healthier alternatives.

For most children, the best source of vitamin A is cod liver oil.

The supplements discussed in this section are primarily recommended for use by children and nursing mothers but can also be used by adults of any age. While generally regarded as safe and effective, these non-drug alternatives to vaccines should be used as directed on the labels or as recommended by a natural health care provider. Dosages will vary according to age and other factors, including past medical history, current nutritional status and weight.

Vitamin A

Supplementation with vitamin A has been shown to reduce the severity of measles infections. Vitamin A deficiency increases susceptibility to any infection. For most children, the best source is cod liver oil (one tablespoon or three capsules daily). Adults can take twice this amount, especially if they are prone to infections or exposed often to individuals with flus, colds or other infections. Cod liver oil has the added benefit of the essential fatty acid omega-3, known for its anti-inflammatory benefits.

Vitamin A can only be reliably obtained from animal sources. Fruits, vegetables and other plant sources contain no vitamin A but are high in beta-carotene (pro-vitamin A). The body can usually convert plant source carotene into vitamin A. In some people who are hypothyroid or deficient in zinc, copper, iodine, selenium or the amino acid tyrosine, this conversion does not take place and carotene accumulates, leaving the skin with a yellow-orange pigmentation.

The use of beta-carotene may act to prevent the development of various cancers. Beta-carotene is not toxic to the liver even in high doses. Large doses of beta-carotene increase the body's demands for vitamin E. If you take 50,000 to 100,000 units of beta-carotene per day, increase vitamin E to 1,000 to 2,000 units per day.

Bovine Colostrum

Colostrum is the first mammary secretion that female mammals provide newborns in the first twenty-four to forty-eight hours after birth. It contains numerous immune system and growth factors, which trigger at least fifty processes in a newborn, ranging from the development of the immune system to the growth of all body cells.

Laboratory analysis of immune and growth factors from bovine colostrum are identical to those found in human colostrum, except for the fact that the levels of these factors are significantly higher in the bovine version. Supplementation with this product enhances immunity in children and adults alike.

Fighting viruses with conventional medical approaches are, at best, problematic. Standard vaccinations and antiviral drugs can all cause significant side effects, including death. On the other hand, hundreds of studies indicate that colostrum is a safe and effective agent for both the prevention and treatment of common viral illnesses.

At present, bovine colostrum is available at health food stores or through health care practitioners without prescription. Unfortunately, there are several poor-quality colostrum products on the market that are biologically inactive due to improper

Bovine Colostrum

Conventional medical doctors were, at one time, enthusiastic about using colostrum for antibiotic purposes. This occurred prior to the introduction of sulfa drugs and penicillin. And prior to the wide spread use of corticosteroids as anti-inflammatory agents, colostrum was used for the treatment of rheumatoid arthritis. Dr. Albert Sabin discovered that colostrum contained antibodies against polio and recommended it for children susceptible to catching the disease. Ayurvedic physicians in India have been using bovine colostrum therapeutically for thousands of years.

In the past five years, North American scientists and health care practitioners have rediscovered this natural supplement. Bovine colostrum is gaining prominence because of its myriad preventive applications in humans, a fact that has not escaped the notice of drug manufacturers who have tried to copy (genetically engineer), patent and market several of the individual components of colostrum.

Well-known colostrum components like interferon, gamma globulin, growth hormone, IgF-1 and protease inhibitors are all used by conventional medical specialists in the treatment of cancer, chronic viral infections, HIV and autoimmune disease. There are now over 4,000 clinical studies from around the world detailing research that has been done using colostrum in the treatment of dozens of different diseases.

processing. To get optimal health results from colostrum supplementation, make sure that the brand you purchase is in powdered or encapsulated powder form and is produced organically-free of pesticides, herbicides and anabolic hormones. Purchase a product that originates from USDA-certified manufacturers; this ensures that strict quality-control procedures were adhered to.

Colostrum may well be the only practical protection on the planet against autoimmune disease, cancer and other incurable diseases. It is completely natural, free of side effects and an excellent alternative to hundreds of drugs. If you are worried about vaccinations, aids, hepatitis, herpes, allergies or chronic fatigue syndrome, colostrum is definitely worth your consideration.

Probiotics

Cultured dairy products like yogurt, acidophilus, raw milk, buttermilk, sour cream, cottage cheese and kefir are the best-known sources of friendly bacteria.

Supplementation with probiotic products provides another unique type of protection against most common infections, allergies and cancers. Probiotics is the name given to the"friendly" bacteria that maintain a healthy intestinal flora, an essential aspect of overall health.

Probiotics prevent the overgrowth of undesirable intestinal bacteria and micro-organisms that produce putrefactive and carcinogenic toxins. If harmful bacteria dominate the intestines, essential vitamins and enzymes are not produced, and the level of harmful substances rises, leading to cancer, liver and kidney disease, hypertension and arteriosclerosis.

Well-known probiotics include Lactobacillus acidophilus and Bifidobacterium bifidum. Another probiotic that has recently generated a great deal of interest is the friendly yeast known as Saccharomyces boulardii, an organism that belongs to the brewer's yeast family. S. boulardii is not a permanent resident of the intestine, but taken orally it produces lactic acid and some B vitamins, and has an overall immune-enhancing effect.

Probiotics are considered to be very safe and well tolerated in the usual dosages prescribed. Highly sensitive individuals have reported the occasional occurrence of indigestion (nausea, heartburn) that disappeared when the supplement was discontinued or the brand of probiotic was changed.

Vaccinations, x-rays, prescription antibiotics, steroids, chlorine, tobacco, caffeine, alcohol and sugar inhibit probiotics. There is also some evidence that casein, a milk protein found in most commercial dairy products, inhibits probiotic growth. The antibiotics found in dairy products are also a factor in suppressing probiotics. A diet high in complex carbohydrates (vegetables, fruits, whole grains, legumes) encourages the proliferation of most probiotics.

Nondigestible food factors that selectively stimulate the growth and activity of probiotics in the gut are referred to as "prebiotics." The best example of a prebiotic is FOS (fructo-oligo-saccharides). This substance is found naturally in many vegetables, grains and fruits, including Jerusalem artichokes, chicory, burdock, garlic and onions. In Japan, FOS is widely used as a sweetener.

Cultured dairy products like yogurt, acidophilus milk, buttermilk, sour cream, cottage cheese and kefir are the best-known sources of friendly bacteria. Equally effective probiotic sources include cultured/fermented soy products like soymilk, tofu, tempeh and miso. Other, lesser-known food sources of probiobtics are sauerkraut and sourdough breads. If dietary sources are not easily available, supplemental probiotic powders and capsules are good alternatives.

Larch arabinogalactan

Larch arabinogalactan is found in a wide range of plants, including carrots, radishes, black beans, pears, wheat and tomatoes, but most abundantly in the Larch tree. Immune-enhancing herbs like echinacea also contain significant amounts.

Larch arabinogalactan has very potent immune-enhancing properties and has been approved by the FDA as an excellent source of dietary fiber. Supplementation will lower the generation and subsequent absorption of ammonia, a potent neurotoxin. It also protects colon cells against cancer-promoting agents.

Like colostrum and probiotics, larch arabinogalactan has an array of clinical uses, both in the prevention and treatment of numerous conditions associated with lowered immune function.

As a food supplement, larch arabinogalactan is available in powdered form. It has a very slight pine-like odor and a sweet taste. It mixes very well with any beverage. The usual adult dose is one to three tablespoons daily. Children under age four can easily take one-half teaspoon daily. Both children and adults can take much higher amounts for various medical conditions. It has no significant side effects except for occasional bloating and flatulence. While not yet well documented or studied for its clinical applications, larch arabinogalactan shows a great deal of promise as a natural immunizing agent.

Interferon Boosters . . . .

Interferon can stimulate the immune system to produce more of the disease-fighting T-cells.

Using a combination of vitamins, minerals, herbs and other food factors that increase interferon production can further bolster immunity. Interferon is produced naturally by the body's white cells to fight and prevent viral and other infections, as well as cancer, allergies and toxic poisoning of the body. A fever stimulates the body to make more interferon, one of the reasons why naturopaths are against the use of drugs to suppress fevers. Interferon can stimulate the immune system to produce more of the disease-fighting T-cells.

Many natural substances have been shown to stimulate the body's natural production of interferon. Some of the best known and documented ones are listed here (in alphabetical order):

Astragalus - This Chinese herb enhances antibody reaction to antigens, increases T-lymphocyte activity, improves symptoms of many HIV-related problems and increases the body's production of interferon. In traditional Chinese medicine, astragalus enjoys a long history of use as an immune system booster and potent tonic for increasing energy levels. Astragalus has been proven to enhance immunity in cancer patients and offsets bone marrow suppression and gastrointestinal toxicity caused by chemotherapy and radiation. No side effects have been reported.

Boneset - Native American Indians use this herb successfully for the treatment of colds, flus, coughs, fevers, indigestion and pain. It has antiseptic properties, promotes sweating, is antiviral and boosts the immune system by enhancing the body's own secretion of interferon.

Echinacea (Echinacea angustifolia) - North American Indians have used echinacea as a treatment for toothaches, snake bites, insect bites or stings and all types of infections. It has a reputation as a blood purifier and also has interferon-like properties. It fights both strep and staph infections, candida (yeast infections) and can kill fungi. It has been used successfully for blood poisoning, ulcers, tuberculosis, childhood infections of every kind and a long list of skin, digestive and immune system disorders.

Most herbalists recommend that echinacea be used on an intermittent basis (three weeks on, two weeks off) because its immune-boosting effects wane if used continuously. I do not agree with this. According to a growing number of herbalists like Canada's Dr. Terry Willard, the on-off use of echinacea is unnecessary since studies indicate continued usage is best.

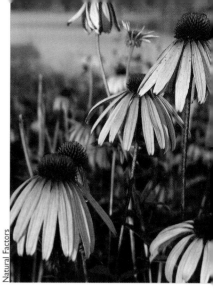

Echinacea has potent immune-stimulatory properties.

Germanium - Many practitioners use this trace mineral for the treatment of chronic fatigue, allergies, infections and cancer. A good source of naturally occurring germanium is Korean ginseng. One's levels of germanium can be determined through hair mineral analysis. If levels are low, supplementation is warranted.

Licorice - Many of the world's cultures have used licorice as a tonic and energy booster, as well as for the treatment of infections and female disorders. Licorice has anti-inflammatory and antiallergic properties. The two licorice components, *glycyrrhizin* and *glycyrrhetinic acid*, stimulate the production of interferon by the body. Licorice is very helpful for coughs, colds and flus, and heals inflamed mucous membranes in the respiratory tract.

Medicinal Mushrooms - Reishi, Maitake, Shiitake, Kombucha, among others, stimulate many aspects of the immune system, including the production of interferon.

Pau D'arco - This herb is well known for its antifungal properties and its stimulating effect on the immune system. Several anecdotal reports have indicated that it could help fight cancer.

Vitamin A and Beta-carotene - Both nutrients boost interferon production. (See page 26.)

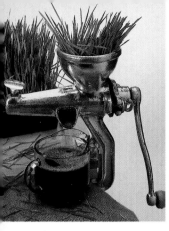

Vitamin C and Bioflavonoids - Vitamins C boosts interferon production. Especially beneficial are pycnogenols like grape seed extract, pine bark extract and bilberry, as well as quercetin, hesperidin and catechin.

Wheat Grass - This "superfood" is rich in vitamins, minerals, amino acids and enzymes. It also enhances interferon production. It is taken in juice form.

Other Natural Immunizing Agents . . .

Oil of Oregano (Origanum vulgare) - This oil is well known in the Mediterranean world for its ability to slow down food spoilage through its antibacterial, antiviral, antifungal, antiparasitic and antioxidant activity. Oregano oil boosts the immune system. It also acts as a free radical scavenger, protecting against toxins and preventing further tissue damage while encouraging healing.

Take two or three drops under the tongue with some olive oil (to improve palatability) several times daily. It is non-toxic and an effective treatment for a variety of conditions.

Colloidal silver - Colloidal silver is both an immune system stimulant and a natural anti-microbial agent. The popularity of colloidal silver is on the rise, especially because of growing concerns over the many hazards of commonly prescribed antibiotic drugs.

Colloidal silver has been documented to contain broad-spectrum germicidal properties, and was used as an antibiotic by doctors before the development of modern antibiotics. The dosages of silver used in the pre-antibiotic era were far in excess of the dosages now recommended.

Recent studies suggest that the relatively dilute colloidal silver products sold without a prescription, lack effective germicidal activity or immune-stimulating effects. Despite these drawbacks, there are hundreds of anecdotal reports about the effectiveness of colloidal silver for a long list of infectious diseases.

Be aware that the long-term use of colloidal silver increases the risk of developing a condition called argyria, whereby excess silver is deposited in the skin and tissues causing

Colloidal silver was used as an antibiotic by doctors before the development of modern antibiotics.

discoloration and skin damage. Colloidal silver could conceivably work well as a homeopathic remedy for a broad range of infectious diseases on a short-term basis.

Homeopathic Nosodes . . . .

Homeopathy is a system of healing developed over 200 years ago by Dr. Samuel Hahnemann. It uses infinitesimally small dosages of natural remedies that rarely have side effects and are well tolerated by adults, the elderly, infants, children and even pregnant women. Several published epidemiological studies suggest that homeopathic remedies are capable of equaling or surpassing standard vaccinations in preventing disease. One report concluded that populations treated homeopathically and then exposed to disease had a 100 percent success rate in preventing that disease.

A certain type of homeopathic remedy called a nosode, made from cultures of microbes and viruses, is most often used as a direct vaccine alternative. The preparation is said to carry the molecular imprint of the proteins and other constituents of the pathological agent. The nosode sensitizes the immune system to this molecular imprint without exposure to the virulence of the living agent.

The administration of a nosode for each of the common childhood diseases is said by homeopaths to be an ideal way to start building immunity. For more information on homeopathic vaccines see *The Vaccine Guide, Making an Informed Choice* by Randall Neustaedter (North Atlantic Books, 1996). For more on nosodes and similar remedies, consult a homeopathic physician.

Several published epidemiological studies suggest that homeopathic remedies are capable of equaling or surpassing standard vaccinations in preventing disease.

33

A Plan of Action . . . .

There are alternatives to conventional immunizations. If you have made the decision to forgo vaccinations for yourself or your child, the next step is to develop a plan of action.

Use the information provided in this book as a guideline, and consult with a health care practitioner who supports your decision and will work with you to implement the changes necessary to minimize susceptibility to disease–the natural way.

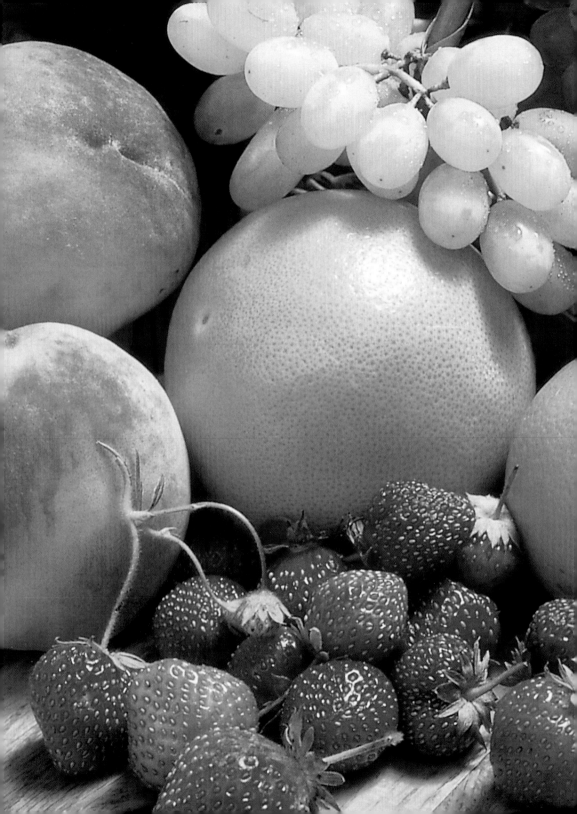

Immune-Boosting Recipes

A whole foods diet is an immune-enhancing diet.

Potato-Mushroom Salad

This tasty pairing of potatoes and mushrooms provides a double dose of immune-boosting nutrients and flavor. The natural chemicals in potatoes protect against viruses, while oyster mushrooms contain the antiviral substance, *lentinan*, which stimulates the immune system.

1 small head romaine lettuce

2 red skin potatoes, cooked with skin

1 tbsp olive oil

1 cup (120 g) oyster mushrooms

1 rosemary branch for garnish

Cherry tomatoes for garnish

Yogurt Mint Dressing

½ cup (150 ml) natural yogurt

2 tsp lemon juice

1 tsp fresh mint, chopped

2 tsp extra virgin olive oil

½ tsp rosemary, chopped

½ tsp dry mustard

Herbamare Vegetable Salt to taste

Thoroughly mix all dressing ingredients together and set aside.

Cut the potato in 1" chunks. Heat 1 tablespoon of olive oil and sauté the oyster mushrooms until golden brown (do not overcook). Remove the mushrooms from the pan and set aside.

Put the cooked potatoes in the pan and sauté for 2 minutes, just to warm them up. Don't let them get brown. Put half of the yogurt dressing in a medium mixing bowl. Add warm potatoes and mushrooms and toss together until everything is covered with the dressing.

Arrange salad on romaine lettuce and drizzle remaining dressing over the salad. Garnish with cherry tomatoes and rosemary.

Serves 2

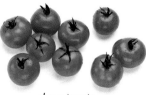

cherry tomato

Herbamare is a seasoning made with sea salt and 14 organic herbs. The special steeping process used to make this natural product allows the full herb and vegetable flavor to become concentrated in the salt crystal–preserving essential vitamins and minerals and providing ultimate zest.

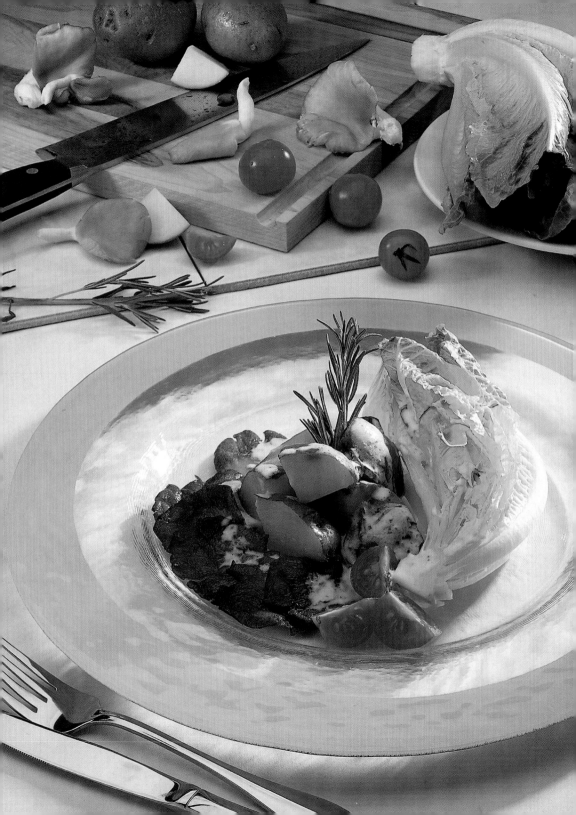

Minestrone with Bow Tie Pasta

1 clove garlic, minced

½ onion, diced

½ cup (150g) **black beans, cooked**

½ cup (100g) **whole wheat bow tie pasta, cooked**

1 cup (150g) **zucchini, cut in ¼" chunks**

1 cup (150g) **broccoli florettes**

½ cup (150g) **yellow bell pepper, cut in ¼" chunks**

½ cup (150g) **red bell pepper, cut in ¼" chunks**

½ cup (150g) **asparagus, cut in ¼" chunks**

½ cup (150g) **Brussels sprouts**

½ cup (150g) **celery, cut in ½" slices**

½ cup (150g) **tomato, cut in ½"chunks**

4 tbsp olive oil

1 bay leaf

1 branch rosemary

1 branch thyme

Herbamare Vegetable Salt to taste

Heat olive oil in a medium sauce pan. Add onion and garlic to the oil and sauté for 1 or 2 minutes. Add remaining vegetables (except for the broccoli and beans) and sauté for 5 minutes. Add vegetable stock, bay leaf, rosemary and thyme and cook for approximately 10 more minutes. Add broccoli, pasta and black beans. Simmer for another 4 to 5 minutes and serve.

Serves 2

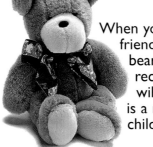

When you see this friendly teddy bear beside a recipe, you will know it is a recipe that children love!

This homemade soup is wonderful with homemade bread. For whole foods bread recipes you can make in your breadmaker read *Healthy Breads with the Breadmaker* (alive Natural Health Guides, 2000).

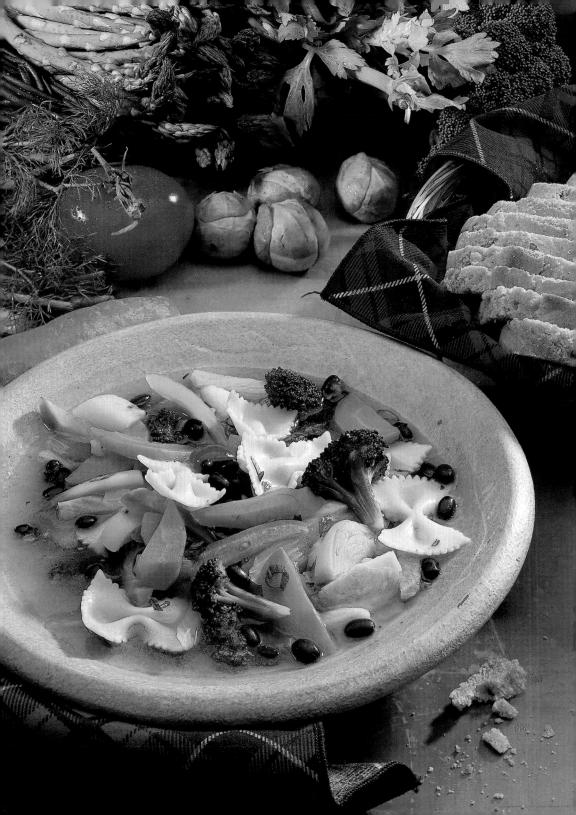

Salad with Jerusalem Artichoke

The wonderful Jerusalem artichoke is often overlooked as an option for a delicious meal. It is rich in minerals—especially iron—and provides a good source of friendly bacteria.

2 cups (150g) green bell pepper

½ cup (100g) Jerusalem artichoke, julienned

1 ripe organic apple, peeled and julienned

1 orange, peeled and cut in segments, save the juice

Dressing:

Juice of half a lemon

2 tbsp cold-pressed flax seed oil

1 tbsp cold-pressed hazelnut oil

½ tbsp cold-pressed pista chio or pumpkin seed oil

1 tsp Bragg's all-purpose seasoning or Maggi

⅛ tsp Herbamare Vegetable Salt, original

½ tbsp nutritional yeast

⅛ tsp Dijon mustard

½ clove garlic, finely grated

Mix all of the dressing ingredients together in a bowl and set aside.

In a medium size bowl add Jerusalem artichoke, apple and orange juice. Add half of the dressing and set aside for approximately 5 minutes. Place the orange segments on each plate, put pepper greens in the center of each plate with the artichoke and apple on top. Drizzle the rest of the dressing on top of the greens.

Serves 2

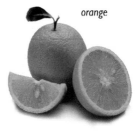

orange

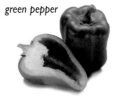

green pepper

Do not toss pepper greens in a bowl as they are very sensitive and delicate.

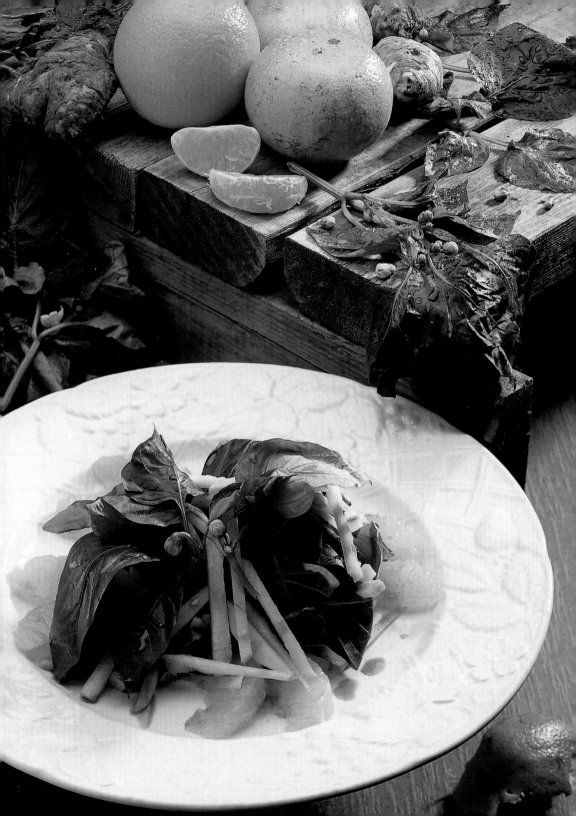

Potato Pancakes with Trio of Greens

Potato Pancakes:

2 lb potatoes, peeled and cooked

½ medium onion, minced

¼ cup (80g) green onions

¼ cup (80g) red bell pepper

¼ cup (80g) yellow bell pepper

4 tbsp olive oil

1 large egg

pinch of nutmeg

1 tsp sea salt

Herbamare Vegetable Salt to taste

Trio of greens:

2 cups (200g) spinach, stems removed

1 lb bok choy, white part of stems removed

2 cups (150g) green bell pepper

4 cloves garlic, minced

½ medium onion, minced

⅛ cup (40g) sun dried cranberries for garnish

1 tsp sea salt

1 tbsp olive oil

Sauce:

⅛ cup (40g) sun dried cranberries

1 cup (4 oz) kefir (or natural sour cream)

¼ cup (80g) walnuts

Potato Pancakes: Place cooked and drained potatoes on a cookie sheet. Dehydrate in oven at 350° Fahrenheit (180° Celsius) for apx. 5 minutes, or until dry. Remove from oven and purée. In the meantime sauté the vegetables with 2 tablespoons of olive oil, until translucent. Drain very well and add to the puréed potatoes. Add egg, flour, nutmeg and Herbamare. Knead until it has the consistecy of dough. Form small balls and press lightly into patties. In a sauté pan fry the patties with the rest of the olive oil until they are golden brown on both sides. Keep warm in the oven.

Trio of greens: In a medium pot add 1½ l water with the salt and bring to boil. Blanch all vegetable greens for about 3 minutes. Strain and rinse well with ice water. In the meantime sauté onion and garlic with 1 tablespoon of olive oil then add the well-drained vegetables. Sauté for 2 minutes.

Sauce: Mix ingredients and drizzle over pancakes and greens. Garnish with cranberries.

Serves 2

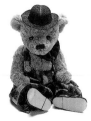

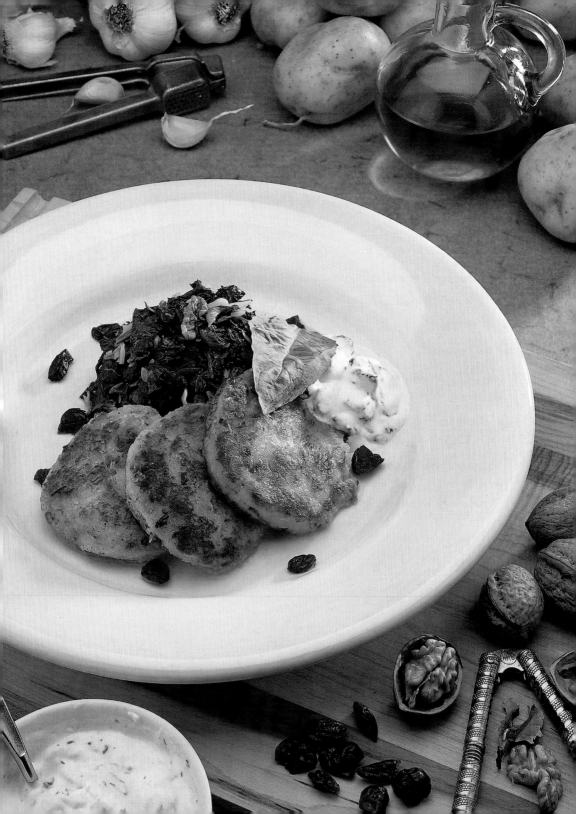

Benoise Omelette

This wonderful omelette makes a nutritious and filling breakfast, lunch or dinner. Served with fresh fruit and whole wheat toast, it is a well-rounded and enjoyable feast.

4 large free-range eggs

¼ cup (80g) red bell pepper, finely chopped

¼ cup (80g) yellow bell pepper, finely chopped

¼ cup (80g) green onion, finely chopped

2 tbsp olive oil

1 large ripe kiwi

¼ cup (80g) strawberries, halved

Segments from one orange for garnish

Herbamare Vegetable Salt to taste

Sauté bell peppers and green onion in the olive oil until translucent. In a medium mixing bowl beat eggs, add Herbamare and pour mixture into the sauté pan with the peppers and onion. (Make sure pan is one that can go into the oven). Carefully fold half of the omelette over the other half. Bake in oven at 300° Fahrenheit (150° Celcius) for 5 minutes. In the meantime place fruit on the plate. Take the omelette out of the oven and serve.

Serves 2

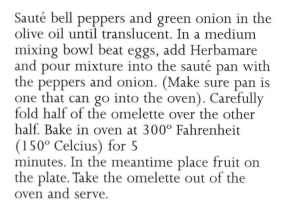

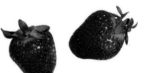

strawberry

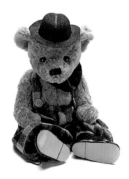

I recommend whole wheat toast, rice milk and a half grapefruit with the omelette.

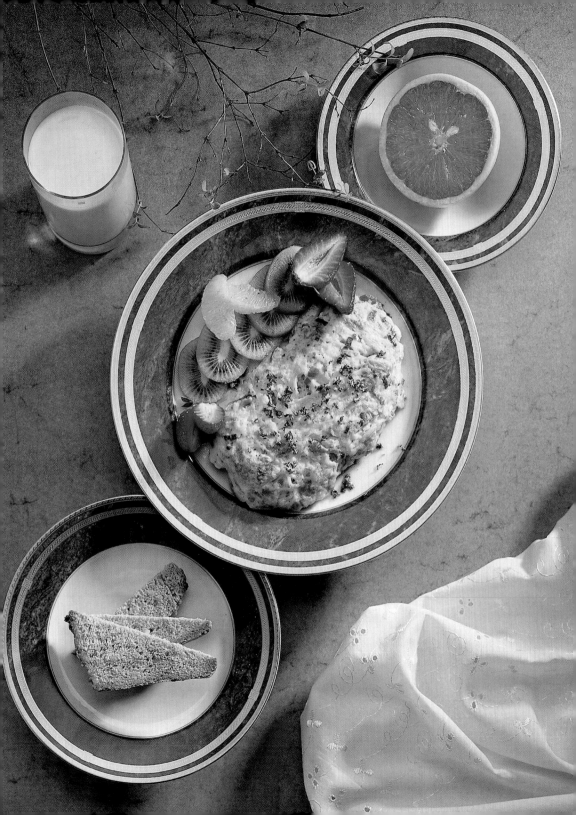

Steamed Vegetable Mix

Vibrant, crisp and teeming with nutrients, this beautiful combination of vegetables provide an immune-boosting and exciting meal.

1 cup (150g) **broccoli florettes**

1 large (100g) **carrot, peeled and sliced in half, lengthwise**

1 cup (100g) **oyster mushrooms**

2 large pieces (100g) **baby bok choy**

1 cup (100g) **soy bean sprouts**

1 large tomato

1 cup (100g) **green turnip, cut in strips**

2 pieces celery, cut in 2" **chunks**

4 oz. (100 g) **Japanese Soba noodles**

2 tbsp black sesame seeds

1 tbsp green onion, **chopped for garnish**

Pinch sea salt

Herbamare Vegetable Salt **to taste**

1 tbsp soy sauce

2 tbsp sesame oil

It is ideal to steam the vegetables in a bamboo steamer. If you do not have this type of steamer any means of steaming will do.

While the vegetables are steaming (which only takes about five minutes) bring a pot with ½ quart (½ l) of water and a pinch of salt to boil. Add Soba noodles and cook for only 2 minutes. Drain and put in a sauté pan with one tablespoon of soy sauce and one tablespoon sesame seed oil. Toss with green onions and black sesame seeds and serve with the steamed vegetables.

Serves 2

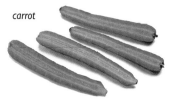

carrot

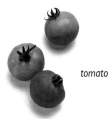

tomato

For a special flavor add two pieces of lemon grass, one piece of ginger or a bay leaf (or any other spice you prefer) to the vegetables while they steam. Don't leave the vegetables unattended when you are steaming them. The cooking process in a bamboo steamer—once the water is boiling—is very fast.

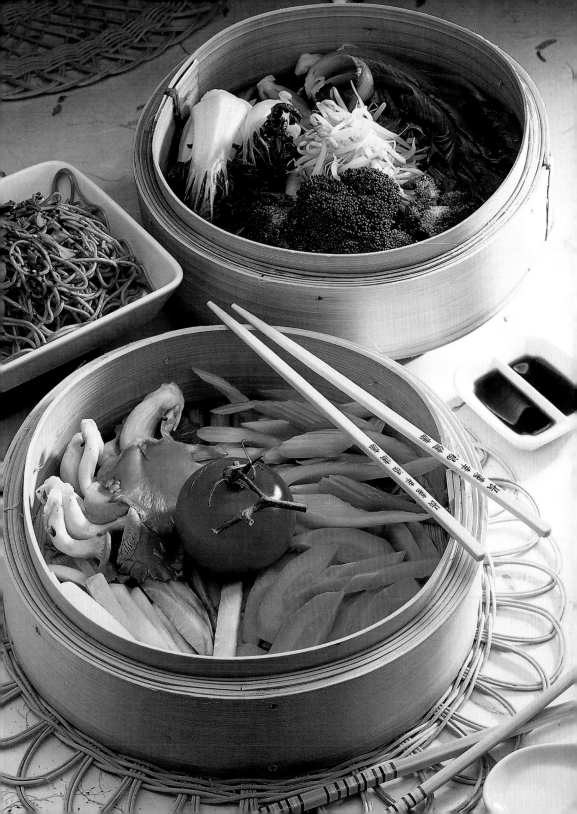

Roasted Potatoes with Poached Eggs

This healthy variation of fried eggs and hash browns is an amazingly tasty way to satisfy hunger, please the taste buds and boost the immune system.

½ lb (apx. 3 small) **Yukon gold potatoes**

½ cup (100g) **green onions, chopped**

2 large free-range eggs

½ tsp sea salt

1 tsp white wine vinegar

1 tsp fresh rosemary, chopped

1 tsp fresh parsley, chopped

4 tsp olive oil or coconut butter

Herbamare Vegetable Salt to taste

Wash, boil, peel and slice potatoes. Sauté potatoes in olive oil or coconut butter, until golden brown on both sides. Season with Herbamare and add green onion and fresh herbs. Meanwhile in a small pot bring ½ quart (½ l) of water to a boil and add salt and vinegar. Crack the eggs into the
boiling water. Cook for 3 to 4 minutes until both the egg white and yolk get slightly firm. Take eggs out of the water with a straining spatula to ensure they are properly drained.

Place the potatoes in the center of the plate and put eggs on top. Serve with a salad of your choice.

Serves 2

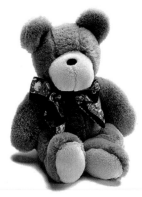

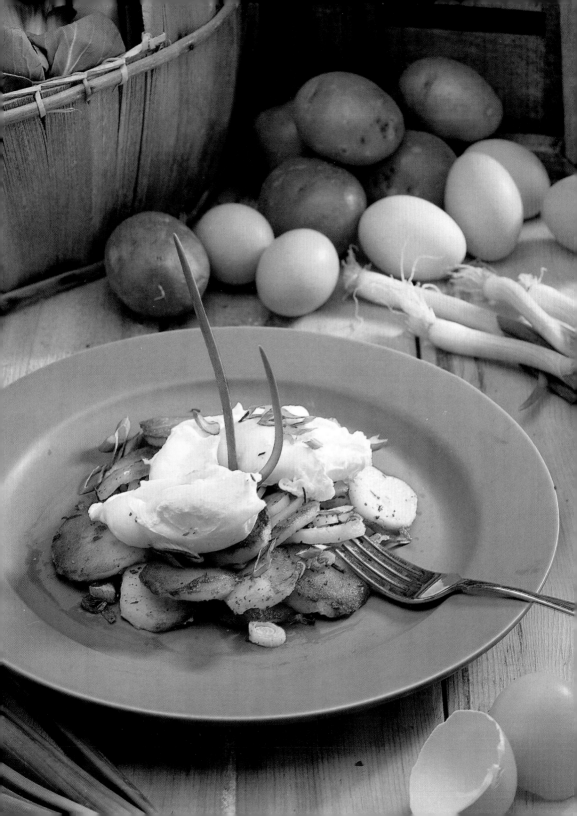

Split Pea Soup

A warm and healthful soup on a cold day eases the mind as well as the stomach. This hearty recipe provides so many immune-boosting ingredients that you may serve it as a complete meal.

I cup (120g) **green split peas, cooked**

I cup (120g) **Yukon gold potatoes, peeled and cut in ½" chunks**

I cup (120g) **turnip, peeled and cut in ½" chunks**

I cup (120g) **carrots, peeled and cut in ½" chunks**

I cup (120g) **onion, diced**

I **clove garlic, diced**

I cup (120g) **celery root, peeled and cut in ½" chunks**

2 **bay leaves**

I **tsp turmeric**

I **rosemary stem**

2 **tbsp olive oil**

⅔ **quart (⅔ l) vegetable stock**

Herbamare Vegetable Salt to taste

Cook split peas in ½ quart (½ l) of water for 15 minutes, or until soft. Set aside. Sauté onion, garlic and all of the vegetables in olive oil until tender. Add turmeric and bay leaves. Add vegetable stock and split peas and bring to boil. Cook for 4 to 5 minutes and then reduce heat to medium. Simmer for another 5 minutes and add rosemary. Season with Herbamare and serve.

Serves 2

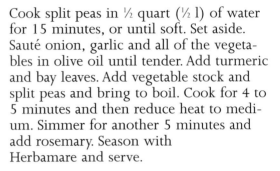

garlic

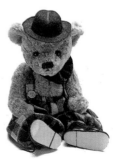

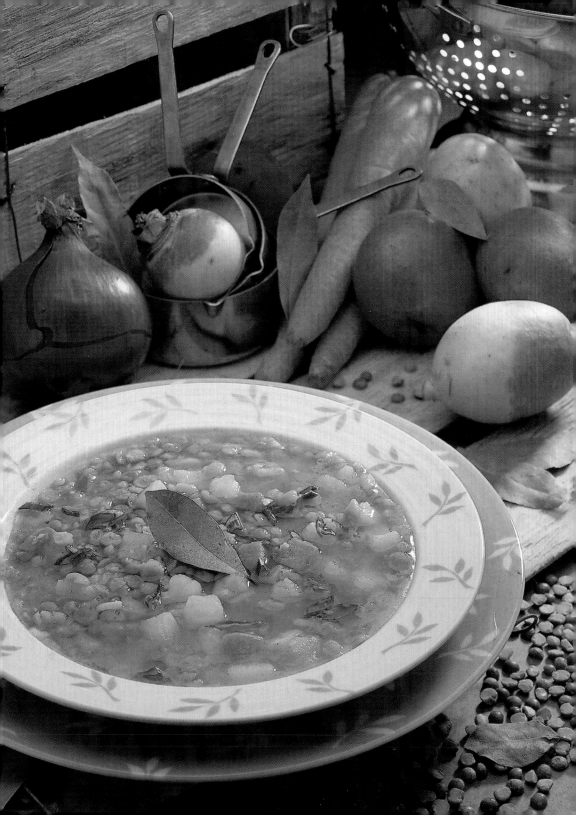

Stir Fried Veggies in a Rice Blanket

½ cup (120g) **uncooked basmati rice**

2 pieces rice paper, 8" diameter (available in Asian grocery store)

2 cups (480ml) **water**

1 tsp sea salt

1 tbsp green onion, chopped

1 tsp black sesame seeds

1 cup (120g) **cauliflower florettes**

1 cup (120g) **broccoli florettes**

1 cup (120g) **red bell pepper, cut in 1" diamond shapes**

1 cup (120g) **yellow bell pepper, cut in 1" diamond shapes**

1 cup (120g) **carrots, cut in 1" slices**

1 cup (120g) **snow peas**

½ **cup** (80g) **green onions, chopped**

½ **cup** (60ml) **toasted sesame seed oil**

½ **cup** (60ml) **soy sauce**

1 tsp fresh cilantro, chopped

Herbamare Vegetable Salt to taste

Bring salt and 1 cup water to boil and add rice. Stir and cook until liquid is reduced by ⅓. Add black sesame seeds and green onion and cook slowly at medium heat until all liquid is evaporated. Set aside. In the meantime soak the rice paper in luke warm water and drain well. Place 2 to 3 tablespoons of cooked rice in the center of the rice paper and fold like a cushion. Place in a frying pan and in one tablespoon of olive oil, or organic cold-pressed canola oil, fry both sides until golden brown and crisp. Keep warm. In the meantime blanch all vegetables in boiling water for 2 minutes. Drain well and rinse in ice cold water. In a wok or sauté pan, heat up the sesame seed oil and toss the vegetables. Add soy sauce, cilantro and Herbamare. Toss well, once again. Place the vegetables in the center of a plate and one rice cushion on top.

Serves 2

A very attractive way to wrap the cushion like a bundle is with two strings of green onion or leek. Blanch the strings in hot water for one or two minutes. This prevents them from breaking or ripping.

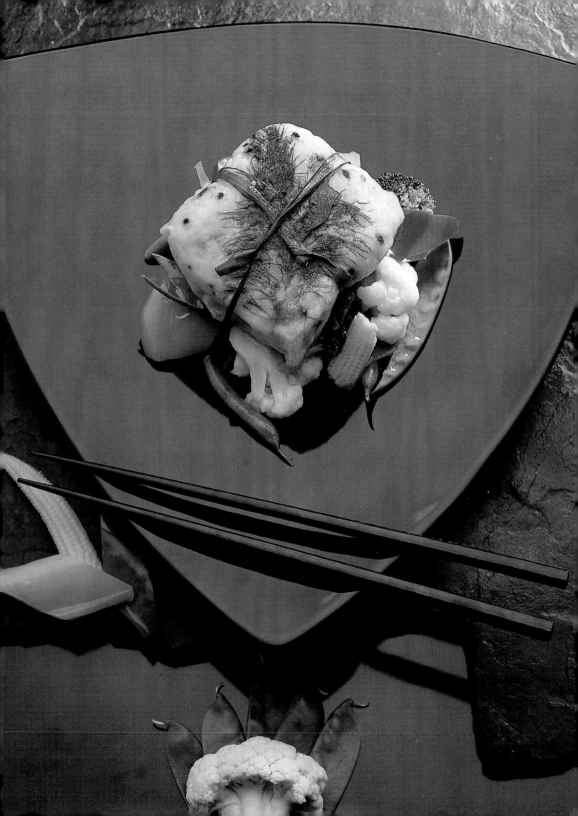

Fennel-Apple Gratin

2 fennel bulbs (450g), **finely julienned**

2 large organic apples (250g), **finely julienned**

2 medium size yam (250g), **peeled, cooked and cut in strips**

I cup (120g) **leeks, finely julienned**

½ cup (100g) **walnuts**

½ cup (120ml) **kefir**

½ tsp nutmeg

I tsp fresh thyme, chopped

2 tbsp olive oil

I tsp maple syrup

Salt and pepper to taste

Yogurt Sauce:

½ cup (100 g) **whole wheat flour**

I cup (225 ml) **yogurt**

I free-range egg

I tbsp olive oil

2 tbsp water

In a large pan, with 1 tablespoon olive oil, gently sauté fennel, apple and leek at medium heat until translucent. Add walnuts, kefir, nutmeg and thyme. Sauté for 3 minutes until all ingredients are nicely combined. Put mixture into a casserole dish and bake in oven at 350° Fahrenheit (180° Celsius) for 20 to 25 minutes.

In the meantime, boil yam until tender, drain well and slice in ½" slices. In a small pan combine 1 tablespoon olive oil and maple syrup and glaze the yam slices with the mixture. Arrange yam on plates and serve with a scoop of fennel-apple gratin.

Yogurt Sauce: This yogurt sauce makes a nice crispy crust for your creation. Heat the flour, olive oil and water. Beat the egg and add it to the yogurt. Add the yogurt and egg mixture to the flour mixture and stir with a wooden spoon until it thickens. Serves 2

walnut

When buying yams for this favorite recipe, be sure to choose the darker ones. The darker orange coloring of the yam indicates a higher concentration of disease-fighting cartenoids (phytonutrients).

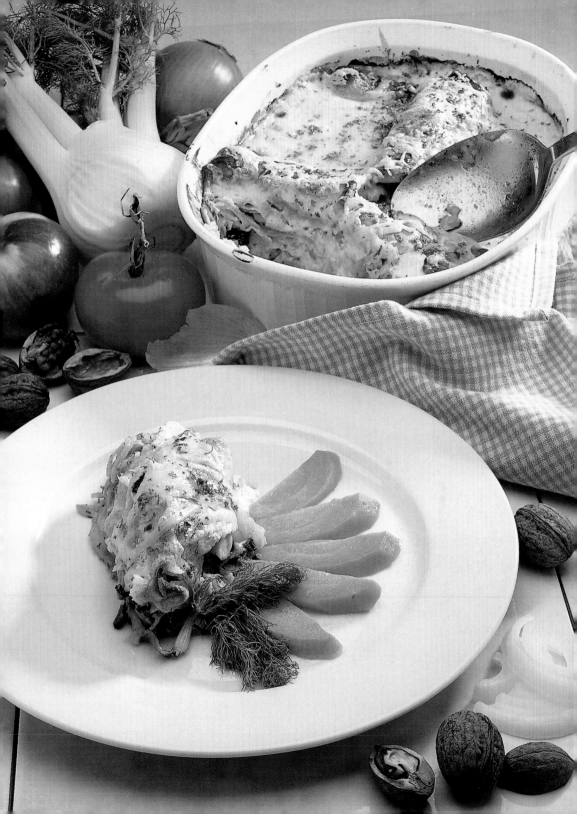

Spaghetti with Artichoke

200 g spaghetti

2 tbsp basil pesto
(see recipe below)

½ cup (100g) green olives

**½ cup (100g) sun dried
black olives**

**½ cup (120g) cherry
tomatoes**

**½ cup (120g)
artichoke hearts**

**½ cup (100g)
oyster mushrooms**

**1 tsp fresh herbs
of your choice**

2 tbsp olive oil

3 tbsp kefir

3 tbsp pasta water

Herbamare Vegetable Salt to taste

In a large pot bring 1½ quarts (1½ l) water and 1 teaspoon salt to boil. Add the pasta to the boiling water and cook until "al dente." Save some pasta water and then drain. Drizzle a couple drops of oil over pasta so that it doesn't stick together. Meanwhile sauté onion, garlic, oyster mushrooms and artichoke hearts in olive oil until tender. Add olives, kefir, pesto and pasta water to the pan. Add pasta, cherry tomatoes and fresh herbs and toss well.

Serves 2

"Al dente" is Italian and means cooked, but still firm to the bite.

Basil Pesto

½ cup (250 g) pine nuts

**3 lbs (1.3 kg) fresh basil
leaves**

**¼ cup (120 g) garlic cloves,
chopped**

**1 cup (250 ml) extra-virgin
olive oil**

1 tbsp sea salt

**1 tbsp freshly ground
pepper**

Heat a cast-iron saucepan and roast the pine nuts until they are golden brown. Wash and dry the basil thoroughly then place in a food processor along with the garlic and pine nuts. Turn food processor on and slowly add olive oil until you get a thick, creamy sauce. Add the salt and blend again.

Leftover Basil Pesto should be frozen.

Never cook fresh basil as it will turn black and taste bitter.

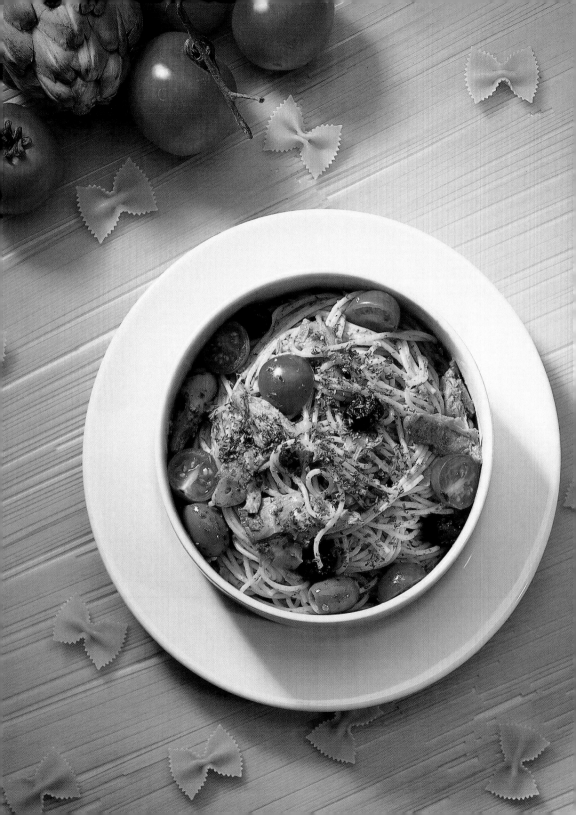

Stuffed Spaghetti Squash

A colorful symphony of taste and nutrition, this immune-boosting recipe is an elegant way to improve health.

- **1 medium (2½-3 lb) spaghetti squash**

- **1 cup (120g) broccoli florettes, blanched**

- **1 cup (120g) cauliflower, blanched**

- **½ cup (100g) Brussels sprouts, blanched**

- **½ cup (100g) red bell pepper, cut in ½" diamond shapes**

- **½ cup (100g) yellow bell pepper, cut in ½" diamond shapes**

- **½ cup (100g) snow peas**

- **½ cup (80g) green onions, chopped**

- **2 tbsp olive oil**

- **1 tbsp flax seed oil**

- **Herbamare Vegetable Salt to taste**

Wash the squash, cut a rectangle (4" long and 2½" wide) in the top of the squash and remove it. Take the seeds out and season the inside of the squash with salt and pepper. Brush the inside of the squash with 1 tablespoon of olive oil. Put the cap back on the squash and bake it in the oven at 400° Fahrenheit (200° Celsius) for 40 to 45 minutes.

In the meantime, bring 1½ quarts (1½ l) of water and 1 teaspoon of salt to boil in a medium pot. Add all the vegetables and blanch for 3 to 4 minutes. Strain them, rinse in ice water and set aside. Take the squash out of the oven and, with a fork, scrape the inside flesh out. In a sauté pan warm up the vegetables and the squash flesh together, with 1 tablespoon of olive oil. Add Herbamare. Add green onion and stuff the vegetables into the squash.

Serves 2

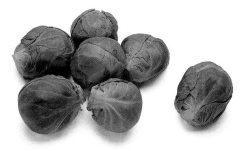

Brussels sprout

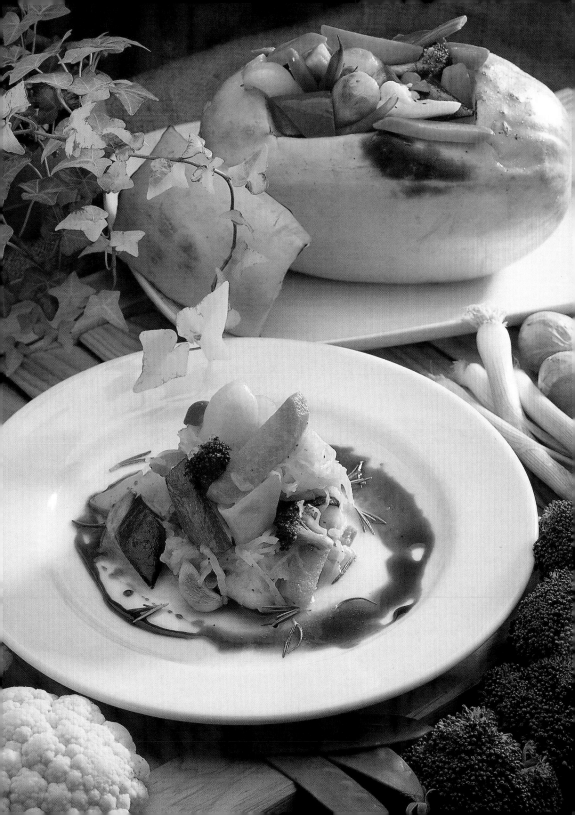

Poached Leek with Mushroom

3 tbsp white wine vinegar

½ tsp sea salt

2 medium leeks

½ cup (200 g) dill pickles, cut lengthwise into ½" (1 cm) pieces

1 cup (300 g) mushrooms, quartered

Tomato Salsa for garnish

¼ cup (60 ml) balsamic vinegar

In a large pot, add vinegar, salt and 2 quarts (2 l) water and bring to a boil.

In the meantime, remove two long leek leaves (use the green part only) to use as strings. Cut the rest of the leek into 2" (5 cm) pieces. Blanch the leek leaves and pieces in boiling water for 4 to 5 minutes. Set aside.

In a large bowl, toss the pickles, mushroom and leek with the balsamic vinegar then arrange in a tower on each plate. Tie together with the poached leek strings. Garnish with Tomato Salsa and serve.

Serves 2

Tomato Salsa

4 small firm Roma tomatoes, diced

¼ red onion, chopped

4 tbsp extra-virgin olive oil

2 tbsp freshly squeezed lime juice

1 tbsp cilantro, chopped

1 tbsp red bell pepper, chopped

1 tbsp yellow bell pepper, chopped

1 tsp garlic, minced

1 small jalapéno pepper, minced

Sea salt, to taste

In a bowl, combine thoroughly all the ingredients. Let sit for at least 2 hours before serving in order for the flavors to incorporate.

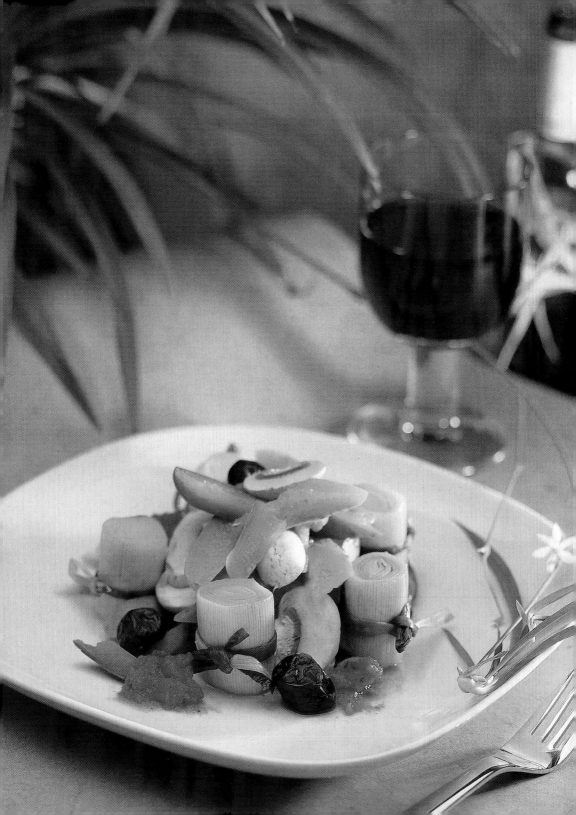

Vegetable Tortellini

Steaming with flavor, this delicious soup provides a wide range of nutrients helpful in maintaining health and boosting the immune system.

1 cup (150g) **vegetable tortellini, cooked**

1 cup (120g) **carrots, diced in ½" cubes**

1 cup (120g) **zucchini, diced in ½" cubes**

1 cup (120g) **leeks, sliced**

1 cup (120g) **celery, cut in ½" chunks**

1 cup (120g) **parsley root, cut in ½" chunks**

½ cup (100g) **onion, diced**

2 cloves **garlic, minced**

1½ quarts (1½ l) **organic vegetable stock** (or water)

2 tbsp **olive oil**

1 tsp **fresh parsley, chopped**

Herbamare Vegetable Salt to taste

In a large saucepan heat olive oil slightly and sauté onion and garlic first and then the rest of the vegetables for 3 to 4 minutes. Add vegetable stock to the saucepan and bring to boil. Cook for 4 to 5 minutes. Add rest of ingredients and simmer on low heat for 3 to 4 minutes.

Serves 2

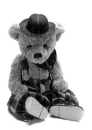

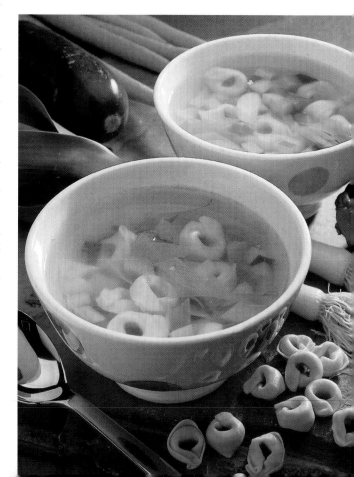

sources

Association For Vaccine-Damaged Children — Manitoba
67 Shier, Winnipeg, MB,
Canada, R3R 2H2.
Tel: 204-895-9192.

Association For Vaccine-Damaged Children — Ontario
116 Ashhurst Crescent
Hampton, ON, Canada, L6V 3N9
Tel: 416-454-2237.

Campaign Against Fraudulent Medical Research
Coordinator: Mr. John Leso
P.O. Box 234 Lawson,
NSW 2783 AUSTRALIA
phone/fax: 61 (047) 58-6822
email: cafmr@pnc.com.au
(CAMFR Canberra: P.O. Box 1327, Woden ACT 2606)

Committee Against Compulsory Vaccination
201 Harbord Street
Toronto, ON, Canada, M5S 1HG
Tel: 416-537-9499.

Center for Empirical Medicine
Harris L. Coulter, Ph.D., Founder
4221 45th Street N.W.
Washington, D.C. 20016, USA.
ph (202) 364 0898
fax (202) 362 3407
email: emptherapies@earthlink.net
Web Page: http://home.earthlink.net/
~emptherapies/

Global Vaccine Awareness League
11875 Pigeon Pass Rd. #B-14-223
Moreno Valley, CA 92557
909-247-4910
Web Page: http://pages.prodigy.com/gval/
email: DQSA45A@prodigy.com

Health Action Network Society
202-5262 Rumble St.
Burnaby, BC V5J 2B6
(604) 435-0512
www.hans.org

Homeopathic Educational Services
2036 Blake St.
Berkeley, CA 94704
orders: 800-359-9051,
fax 510-649-1955
inquiries/catologues 510-649-0294
email: mail@homeopathic.com
Web Page:
http://www.homeopathic.com/index.html

National Vaccine Information Center
512 Maple Avenue West, #206
Vienna, VA 22180
703-938-DPT3; 800-909-7468
email: info@909shot.com
Web Page: http://www.909shot.com

PROVE(Parents Requesting Open Vaccine Education)
P.O. Box 1071
Cedar Park, TX 78630-1071
(512) 918-8760
Email prove@swbell.net (email)
Website: home.swbell.net/prove

Vaccine Information & Awareness (VIA)
Karin Schumacher, Director
792 Pineview Drive
San Jose, CA 95117
408-397-4192 (voice mail/pager)
408-554-9053 (phone/fax)
email: via@access1.net
Web Site: http://www.access1.net/via

Vaccination Risk Awareness Network
439 Wellington St., Suite 5
Toronto, ON, Canada, M5V 1E9
Tel: 416-280-6035.
(VRAN News is published quarterly.)

Vaccines & Alternatives
485 Montford Drive
Dollard-Des-Ormeaux, QB, Canada, H9G 1M7
Tel: 514-483-2959.

Vaccine Awareness Network, NSW (VAN)
Coordinator: Meryl Dorey
P.O. Box 177
Bangalow, NSW 2479
AUSTRALIA
phone: (066) 871-699;
fax: (066) 872-032
email: van@om.com.au

First published in 2000 by
alive books
7436 Fraser Park Drive
Burnaby BC V5J 5B9
(604) 435–1919
1-800–661–0303

© 2000 by **alive** books

Book Design:
 Paul Chau
Artwork:
 Terence Yeung
 Raymond Cheung
 Liza Novecoski
Food Styling/Recipe Development:
 Fred Edrissi
Photography:
 Edmond Fong (recipe photos)
 Siegfried Gursche
Photo Editing:
 Sabine Edrissi-Bredenbrock
Editing:
 Sandra Tonn
 Marian Maclean

Canadian Cataloguing in Publication Data

Rona, Zoltan
 Natural Alternatives to Vaccination

(**alive** natural health guides, 7
ISSN 1490-6503)
ISBN 1-55312-009-4

Printed in Canada

Revolutionary Health Books

alive Natural Health Guides

Each 64-page book focuses on a single subject, is written in easy-to-understand language and is lavishly illustrated with full color photographs.

New titles will be published every month in each of the four series.

Self Help Guides	**Healthy Recipes**	**Healing Foods & Herbs**	**Lifestyle & Alternative Treatments**
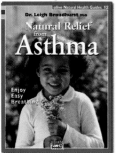	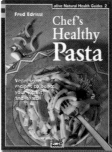	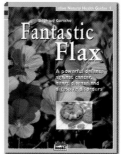	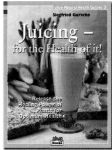

Self Help Guides

Healthy Recipes

Healing Foods & Herbs

Lifestyle & Alternative Treatments

other titles to follow:

other titles to follow:

other titles to follow:

other titles to follow:

Self Help Guides
- **Natural Treatment for Chronic Fatigue Syndrome**
- **Fibromyalgia Be Gone!**
- **Heart Disease: Save Your Heart Naturally**
- **Liver Cleansing Diet**

Healthy Recipes
- **Baking with the Bread Machine**
- **Chef's Healthy Salad**
- **Healthy Breakfasts**
- **Desserts**
- **Smoothies and Other Healthy Drinks**

Healing Foods & Herbs
- **Calendula: The Healthy Skin Helper**
- **Ginkgo Biloba: The Good Memory Herb**
- **Rhubarb and the Heart**
- **Saw Palmetto: The Key to Prostate Health**
- **St. John's Wort: Sunshine for Your Soul**

Lifestyle & Alternative Treatments
- **Maintain Health with Acupuncture**
- **The Complete Natural Cosmetics Book**
- **Kneipp Hydrotherapy at Home**
- **Magnetic Therapy and Natural Healing**
- **Sauna: Your Way to Better Health**

Vancouver
Canada

Great gifts at an amazingly affordable price **$9.95 Cdn / $8.95 US / £8.95 UK**

alive Natural Health Guides are available in health and nutrition centers and in bookstores.
For information or to place orders please dial 1-800-663-6513